Alkaline Diet

Quick And Simple Alkaline Diet Recipes For Detox And Rapid Weight Loss

(The Detailed Guide To Understanding PH)

Leonard Hernandez

TABLE OF CONTENT

Delisiouslu Alkalizing Smoothie Resires

Alkalinizing smoothies are a quick and easy method to fill your stomach with as many fresh fruits and vegetables as you desire. The best breakfast or refreshment is prepared for when hunger strikes throughout the day.

They are rich in oluble plant fber, which benefits your entire digestive system, keeps you feeling satisfied, and helps you fight free radicals, in addition to providing numerous vitamins, minerals, phytonutrients, and healing compounds.

Consider whipping up a large batch of smoothie in the morning, pouring it into a stainless steel bottle, and bringing it with you to enjoy throughout the day - there is less need to concern about deterioration with smoothies than with juices. Although theu always taste best fresh, they are still delicious after two hours.

You will notice that all the trees in the book are actually green and smooth. The beet greens are, without a doubt, one of the best food choices you can make for restoring your body's optimal rH levels. Don't let this discourage you; these sombnaton are absolutely delicious. You are free to decrease or increase the amount of green you use for your reference. You may consult the AlkalineFood entry on the primary Alkaline page. Det book to get more ideas for the green foliage vegetables and fruits you can enjoy in your alkalinizing smoothies.

FOR AND AGAINST

PROS Can be satisfying and filling Encourages the consumption of fresh produce

CON Many rules to remember Limited research to correct slam

The alkaline diet encourages increased consumption of fruits and vegetables while discouraging the consumption of foods high in sugar and saturated fat. Increasing fruit and vegetable consumption while decreasing red meat consumption would be advantageous for everyone. The Western diet is low in fruits and vegetables and high in carbohydrates and fat. However, the alkali metal has several disadvantages.

PRO A diet rich in fruits and vegetables is extremely filling, making it easier to complete tasks. While there is no doubt that consuming fewer processed foods is beneficial, there is little evidence to support the claim that alkaline diets affect blood rH for the purpose of treating disease.

It's important to note, however, that the rH levels of the body's tissue areas vary greatly, whereas the rH levels of the entire body remain within a narrow range due to the function of our kidneys and lungs.

CONS

There is no scientific evidence to support the claim that an alkaline diet can improve health or that eating acidic foods can alter the body's pH. For example, diet proponents assert that a high-sodium diet increases the risk of osteoporosis and fractures in older individuals. The theoru the bodu leeshe salsum — an alkalne ubtanse — was extracted from bone to balance out the asdtu. The research, however, does not contradict this. In a 202 10 study, researchers observed 862 men and women aged 70 and found that dietary acid load had no correlation with bone mineral density or osteoporosis diagnosis. Although the diet encourages the consumption of healthful foods, it also encourages the consumption of nutritious foods such as milk and dairy products, which are excellent sources of protein and calcium. The diet's claims about restricting these foods are unfounded, as research indicates that doing so has no adverse effect on the body and does not interfere with sodium metabolism. Is Alkaline Diet a Healthy Option for You?

The alkaline diet emphasizes consuming fresh, whole foods, including a variety of fruits and vegetables, with limited amounts of processed foods. It permits small amounts of animal protein and fat while reducing refined cereals, thereby providing a wide range of nutrients. Dietary guidelines issued by the United States Department of Agriculture (USDA) include calorie and nutrient recommendations for a healthy, well-balanced diet. The USDA recommends the following nutritionally dense foods.7 Vegetables and dark, leafu greens (e.g., kale, srinash, brossoli, Swiss shard, green beans)

Fruits (e.g., arrles, berries, melon)

Grains (such as quinoa, brown rice, and oats)

Lean meats (e.g., shisken breast, fish, turkeu breast)

Bean and legume (such as all beans, lentils, and radish)

Nuts and seeds, such as walnuts, almonds, and sunflower seeds.

Daru (e.g., low-fat milk, kefir, yogurt)
Oils (e.g., olive oil, avocado oil)
Adopting a plant-based diet rich in fruits and vegetables may assist you in achieving overall health and protecting against certain diseases. However, the acid-forming foods on the alkaline diet are rich in fiber, vitamins, and minerals that are essential to good health. These foods include grains, beans, and nuts. In the meantime, the diet includes coffee and wine, which nutrition experts agree should be consumed in moderation.The USDA's dietary guidelines indicate that the number of calories a person needs to meet nutritional requirements and maintain a healthy weight varies based on age, physical activity, and gender. Use this calculator to determine your dietary requirements. The alkalne diet allows for the consumption of all of the foods recommended by the USDA, despite restricting certain amounts of grains, legumes, animal protein, and dairy, and is therefore not necessarily considered healthful as it may lack a variety of nutrients and balance.

What Is An Alkaline Diet?

The alleged antacid diet depends on a body fermented by foods such as white flour, cheddar, meat, eggs, sugar, coffee, and alcohol. The optimal pH range for the human body is between 6.2 and 6.8 in the morning and 6.8 and 7.8 in the evening. A robust climate has a marginally fundamental (antacid) value. The scale of sharpness ranges from 0 to 2 8 , with 0 representing the most basic corrosiveness and 2 8 representing the most exalted essential response; 7 is the most neutral point and corresponds to pure water, i.e. the equilibrium is established. These food sources are generally disapproved of in this diet, so they may only be consumed in small quantities. The ratio of base to acid is reflected in a revised 70:6 0 diet.

A fundamental diet, or even a basic diet, is contingent upon a complete diet change that must be kept up intermittently; thus, it is not a typical diet. 70% of the permitted essentials consist of fundamental food sources such as organic products, vegetables, nuts, and soy products, while 6 0% consist of acidic products.

This diet was conceived by nutritionist Vicki Edgson and chef Natasha Cortt. It was believed that an overly fermented body would become unwell more quickly and that a transcendently basic diet could prevent depression, cardiovascular disease, osteoporosis, and even disease. Natasha Corrett says, "When the body is in its natural state, it functions better; you have more energy, you sleep better, you can concentrate better, your skin is better, your eyes are more beautiful, and your hair is growing faster." In addition, disease cells avoid an essential environment.

It has been established that resveratrol, which is present in red grapes, inhibits angiogenesis by 60%.

Additionally, ellagic acid is primarily found in raspberries and pomegranates (or pure pomegranate juice). Listed below are various food varieties that may have an antigenic effect:

Green Tea

Blackberries, strawberries, raspberries, blueberries

Cherries

Orange, grapefruit, lemon

Muscoda

Ay

Chou kale

Artichokes

Curcuma

Persil

Maitake mushrooms
These dietary varieties contain a variety of potentially antigenic compounds.

Few food sources are significantly more compelling than current antiangiogenic medications. They contain both parsley and garlic.

Consequently, the outcome is more straightforward when these mixtures are taken together, in whole natural product, than when they are taken separately; consequently, it is important to favor a diet that promotes whole food sources, natural rather than remaining fixated on individual nutrients.

Additionally, it is essential to recognize that fructose prejudice may increase the risk associated with this type of sugar.

HOW TO APPLY

nutrients acidifying and alkalizing

The PRAL file is used to quantify whether food is acidifying or alkalizing. This record is computed by separating acidifying minerals (chlorine, sulfur, and phosphorus) from basifying minerals (potassium, magnesium, and calcium) and taking into account the quantity of minerals and their absorption in the intestines.

If PRAL is below 0, the food is alkaline. If PRAL is greater than 0, the food is acidifying.

List of substances that are acidic:

Lactic compounds

Animal products

Cereal products

Sweet confections

Products of processing

Legumes

List of cuisines with a base:

The plant foods

The results

Fruits rich in oleic acid (olive, avocado, coconut)

Aromatic flora and a few medicinal

Coconut, rapeseed, and olive oils
However, there may be exceptions for a few food sources, and in both cases: Citrus fruits (lemon, citrus, etc.).
Their PRAL file is below 0; therefore, on paper, they are alkalizing. Nevertheless, they can ferment given our ability to utilize these acidic food varieties in the mouth. Simply put, if your sensory system is compromised, you will experience chills; if you have chilly tolerance, it is best to avoid these foods. In any case, you should observe your body's reactions following consumption.
Citrus fruit and other fruits
Fruits cause the body to detoxify, resulting in the release of numerous acids. The corrosive-base equilibrium can be disrupted, and as evidenced by our capacity to dispose of these acids, the soil can become noxious relatively quickly. Therefore, it is essential to gradually increase the amount of natural products in the body's systems

and to assist its emunctories (stomach, lungs, kidneys, skin, and liver) in eliminating waste.

Oil-bearing seeds (almonds, cashews, etc.)

They are acidifying (with the possible exception of almonds), but essential for a healthy balance of unsaturated lipids and cell reinforcement. Their usage should be restricted to a few small clusters per day. Be sure to soak vegetables prior to consuming them to eliminate nutrient-destroying organisms (2 2 hours for almonds, 8 hours for pistachios).

Tomatoes

It is an antacid diet, but the effect on citrus depends on your metabolic rate. Observe your responses. Moreover, note that tomatoes are exceptionally rich in lycopene, a substance that prevents cancer.

Eggs (egg yolk vs. egg white)

Different sources indicate that egg yolk is extremely acidic, despite claims to the contrary. Everyone acknowledges that egg white is acidifying. If you have a reliable source, feel free to send it to me. Despite being neutral or fundamental sugars (PRAL = 0), they are considered acidifying. Certainly, their assimilation intentionally produces acids, which, as a result of oxygenation of the tissues, are transformed and eliminated as water and CO_2. Hence the significance of ensuring adequate oxygenation and facilitating the micronutrient-induced transformation processes. If possible, avoid white or processed carbohydrates that lack essential nutrients and have a high glycemic index - elaboration on which sugar to choose for cookery.

Chocolate

Assuming it is dark and contains somewhere between 70 and 80% cacao, chocolate has a low acridity (PRAL between 0 and 2) by the piece. However, it is an effective "anti-stress" cuisine so long as its consumption is limited. It facilitates the restoration of corrosive base equilibrium by reducing anxiety and tension. Cocoa is likely the richest substance in polyphenols with cell-reinforcing properties and is known to reduce inflammation, prevent colorectal cancer growth, preserve memory, and protect blood vessel health. For those looking to reduce their sugar intake, maltitol or xylitol-containing chocolates are an option. For those who do not recognize the value of chocolate's energizing effect, carob, which is rich in minerals, is a worthwhile alternative. The decision to consume unprocessed cocoa can be made by individuals who need to avoid added substances or consume copious quantities of chocolate.

Note that cooking modifies dietary supplements (especially vitamins C, B2 , and B9). Similarly, imagine that browning your food (neurotic response) can turn it acidic. Therefore, favor delicate simmering or temperatures below 2 00 ° C.

The acidic supper

To make excellent food decisions, you must first be aware of your needs, or give attention to yourself, your body, your emotions, and your desires. It is equally essential to comprehend the mind-boggling climate where we live and how it affects us daily. This increasing awareness aids in refining our decisions, objectives, and demands. It is essential to remain receptive to changes and mistakes, which are essential learning opportunities. Last but not least, recognize that a soluble dinner is relatively simple; it depends only on standards and food preparation techniques known and perceived to aid in the body's recuperation.

Determine your objectives

All cleansing and remaking processes are dependent on the condition of the sensory system, so adjusting the techniques used to recover your tissues and rebalance your environment will be contingent on its status. If it is weak, cleaning and recovery will be sluggish, and you should adopt a dynamic procedure at the risk of degrading the situation further. First, conduct a comprehensive assessment of your current state of health. You can seek advice, perform a blood test, or test the pH level of your urine with pH paper, but your feelings will likely be the best guide. From there, formulate an objective, determine sub-goals, and develop the techniques necessary to achieve this. Defining what you need to achieve assists with overcoming moments of difficulty or tension, periods in which we lose motivation and revert to old habits more readily.

What Foods Are Allowed on the Alkaline Diet?

In this section, we will examine the foods that are permitted on the Alkaline Diet. Eating solid fundamentally soluble food sources is the way to progress on the Alkaline Diet, which means eating basic debris food varieties (80% of your diet) and generally avoiding corrosive debris food sources (20% of your dietary overall).

Consider sources of corrosive detritus as your Kryptonite. Similar to how kryptonite incapacitated Superman to the point where he couldn't defeat his enemies, corrosive debris food varieties can irritate your body to the point of causing or fueling fundamental medical conditions, making you feel less energized, and possibly putting you at risk for genuine medical conditions in the future and accelerating aging. Not to speak for your benefit, but you have no need for that. You must possess the qualities of Superman, Captain America, and Aquaman. You must be vigorous and robust, fit enough to tackle any task with confidence.

Many of you may be familiar with the concept of alleged nutrients. For those of you who are sick, superfoods are healthy, common food varieties that contain cell reinforcements and other synthetic compounds that can help you combat and prevent disease. According to studies, they can live longer. Any Internet search will reveal some of these nutrients, including mango, coconut, kale, chia, avocado, salmon, and garlic, among others.

Despite the fact that many of you are not yet familiar with the basic debris food varieties, those of you who are will notice that the list of these normal nutrients includes some soluble debris food varieties, namely coconut, avocado, and garlic.

While there are some on there that we would consider corrosive debris, such as salmon, the majority of the debris is non-corrosive.

The point here is that, despite the fact that we may consider antacid debris food sources to be "superfoods" because many of them have been shown to have health benefits that can help us live longer, they are not the same as the superfoods you may have read about online.

These were your fundamental debris dietary sources, and there are a great deal of them. This regimen is not comparable to being incarcerated in a foreign nation. You can without much of a stretch make a dinner plan for the day that will enable you to prepare all of your dinners at home using ingredients purchased from your local supermarket or farmer's market. You could actually dine out if that is important to you. You will have many items to peruse! Next on the list (of the rival group) are the dietary sources of corrosive debris. On the Alkaline Diet, you must limit your consumption of these foods. Acid Ash Dietary Chart

A standard version of the Alkaline Ash Diet states that we should consume 80% antacid debris food types and 20% acidic debris food types, so plan accordingly. Moreover, some individuals may choose to consume an alkaline-only diet.

Top Ten Alkaline Foods You Should Consume Daily

2 - Spinach

Spinach is a nutritious vegetable with numerous health benefits, including its anti-acid properties. This is largely due to the spinach's high chlorophyll content, which acts as an alkalizing agent within the body and restores the pH level to its optimal level. In addition to its alkalizing properties, spinach is loaded with essential vitamins and minerals, including A, C, K, E, B2, magnesium, iron, calcium, folate, manganese, and potassium. Thus, spinach alone can help the body feel comfortable and perform at a superior level. It prevents iron deficiency, coronary disease, signs of aging, malignant growth, muscle weakness, and skin damage. For optimal results, consume roughly one cup of spinach per day, raw, prepared, or blended in a smoothie.

2– Lemons

This may surprise you, as lemons are typically regarded an acidic organic food. In any case, they possess a high degree of solubility. This is due to the fact that the citrus extract in lemons has a solubilizing effect on the body. They aid in cleansing and detoxifying the body by utilizing essential minerals such as calcium and iron. Lemons aid the body in the proper functioning of the digestive and immune systems. In addition, they aid in getting in shape, regulate the heart rate, and protect against cancerous cells. To reap the full benefits of lemons, consume a lemon water mixture first thing in the morning on an empty stomach. Simply combine the juice of one lemon segment with a glass of warm water. Then, at least thirty minutes should pass before ingesting food.

6 – Kale

Kale is yet another remarkable green that should be consumed daily. It has pH-balancing properties as well as detoxification and cell-reinforcing properties. Vitamin A, Vitamin K, Vitamin C, Magnesium, Calcium, Copper, Potassium, Iron, Protein, Phosphorus, and Manganese can be found in kale. It is not surprising that kale has been shown to aid in lowering cholesterol, reducing heart rate, shedding pounds, and reducing the risk of disease, given its many beneficial properties. Consume roughly two servings of kale approximately four times per week to reap all of its health benefits.

8 – Avocados

Avocados are another food source that is rich in essential nutrients and minerals that aid in flushing out harmful toxins and restoring the body's optimal pH level. Therefore, avocados benefit the cardiovascular system, the immune system, the circulatory system, and the digestive system. Because avocados are so beneficial to the body, it is advised to consume them frequently. Try to consume a substantial amount of avocado every day. They are divine and can be incorporated into virtually any dish or cocktail.

Five Wheatgrass

Wheatgrass also facilitates in cleansing the body. In doing so, it also helps protect the liver from toxic substances. Wheatgrass aids in sustaining energy, getting in shape, balancing blood sugar, and combating cancerous cells due to its essential nutrients and minerals, as well as its ability to rid the body of toxic buildup. Wheatgrass can be processed in a variety of ways, including extraction from the plant or purchase in powder form. Consume one to two ounces daily if strained. Add one teaspoon to a glass of water and consume daily if the supplement is in powder form.

6– Celery

Celery is an energizing product that does not receive the credit it deserves. Celery is typically included on the menu of all diets. This is largely due to celery's diuretic properties, which aid the body in eliminating excess fluids. Additionally, celery can eliminate acid in the body and restore the pH to a slightly alkaline level. Celery alone can maintain the body's fundamental state. Consume two to three stalks of celery every day, and your pH level should be readily balanced at 7.8 0.

7- Broccoli

Perhaps the most important substance for maintaining an alkaline pH is broccoli. This is because broccoli contains phytochemicals that alkalize the body, reduce estrogen potency, and increase estrogen metabolism. Additionally, broccoli contains cell reinforcements and tranquil properties.

It can affect the gastrointestinal framework, cardiovascular framework, immune framework, and integumentary framework. This is largely due to the vitamins and minerals found in broccoli, which include Vitamin A, Vitamin K, Vitamin C, Iron, Folate, Protein, Fiber, Manganese, and Potassium. To reap the full benefits of broccoli's healthy properties, consume it at least four times per week. Try steaming or simmering it for optimal results.

Eight Cucumbers

Cucumbers are another food with a high water content that helps the body filter out harmful toxins. They can help restore the pH balance of the body by neutralizing acids. They also aid in reducing irritation within the body. Cucumbers are an excellent source of nutrients and minerals and should therefore be ingested frequently. They are minimal in calories and aid in maintaining the body's hydration. They are an incredible addition to any healthy diet. Cucumbers promote cardiac health, glucose levels, digestion, and weight loss by preventing the accumulation of excess fat. They could actually aid in the fight against malignant cells.

9– Bell Peppers

The chime pepper is an incredibly misjudged delicacy. Not only can ringer pepper help to kill corrosive in the body and elevate the pH level to basic, but it can also aid in reducing anxiety, lowering circulatory pressure, reducing inflammation, and fighting cancer. At least one cup of chiming peppers should be consumed three to four times per week. They may be consumed raw, grilled, barbecued, or roasted.

2 0– Garlic

As with many other items on this list, garlic possesses an abundance of health benefits that extend far beyond restoring the pH balance of the body. Garlic aids in promoting the overall health of the body. It includes Vitamins B2 , B6, and C, as well as Calcium,

Copper, Selenium, and Manganese. It functions as an antibacterial food, antiviral food, cancer-prevention food, and parasite-fighting food. For the benefit of neutralizing the body's acids and restoring the pH level, garlic must be crushed or slashed. Due to the necessity of releasing significant sulfur compounds, this is the case. Daily consumption of two to four fresh garlic cloves will stabilize the pH level in the body.

An alkaline diet can be used to treat conditions associated with blood or urine acidosis, such as kidney stones, urinary tract infections, and osteoporosis.

This information is not sufficiently protected. Many of you embarking on the Alkaline Diet are doing so because you may be struggling with a specific medical condition and you have heard that the Alkaline Diet can assist you in resolving that condition. As we have repeatedly stated in various sections of this book, a variety of medical conditions are directly related to consuming corrosive debris-laden food sources with high calorie counts. Numerous unfavorable conditions in the body push the blood toward acidosis, requiring the body to labor longer than necessary to maintain a homeostasis that is not only normal, but essential for life. Actually, you do not need to be ill in order to benefit from the Alkaline Diet. Numerous individuals choose to follow this diet in order to prevent the onset of future diseases or conditions, such as osteoporosis.

The human body takes extraordinary measures to maintain homeostasis, as certain conditions (which we can summarize as homeostasis) are essential for the body to function normally.

Not only is this a crucial aspect of the Alkaline Diet, but it is also a scientific enigma that even the scientific community does not fully comprehend. While the Alkaline Diet may be exceptional in comparison to other diets, it also shares a number of characteristics with them. Numerous modern regimens function by observing how the body normally operates. For instance, the Intermittent Fasting diet capitalizes on how the human body normally processes food as a result of eons of evolution. The human body has evolved to anticipate fasting (non-eating) periods, which are accentuated by feeding periods. In the absence of food, the body consumes fat from its own fat stores to satisfy its caloric needs. This is an illustration of how a diet can take advantage of how the body normally functions. Indeed, the Alkaline Diet differs little from other diets.

The Alkaline Diet capitalizes on the body's natural desire to maintain homeostasis by facilitating the body in arriving. Since you are assisting your body in this cycle, your body does not have to deal with the confusion of acid ash foods flooding the bloodstream when you are already acidotic; now your body not only has to digest these heavilyprocessed acid ash foods, but it also has to attempt to move your circulatory system toward alkalinity, and god forbid you have a kidney stone... In essence, a diet high in corrosive detritus food sources is harmful to the body, especially if you are older, overweight, or have preexisting medical conditions. Homeostasis is a state that your body goes to great lengths to achieve, but you can be a brother and aid it along a bit.

A simple way to conceptualize the Alkaline Diet is to view it as a way to assist the body in achieving homeostasis by avoiding the typically acidic food sources of the Western diet and consuming food types that shift the body away from acidosis.

The purpose of this "secret" is to help you comprehend why the Alkaline Diet is more than a diet; it's a way of life. This diet is not simply a way for you to lose weight or achieve a certain goal. The Alkaline Diet is a method for helping your body function normally, decreasing your risk for future medical conditions, increasing your vitality, and possibly extending your life.

Secret No. 8: The Alkaline Diet can be used to prevent osteoporosis in older individuals by reducing blood acidosis, thereby preventing the body from processing bone and promoting bone deposition.

Old-fashioned osteoporosis. Our dear buddy. The reason we continue to discuss this condition is because it is arguably the greatest example of how the Alkaline Diet can transform individuals. It is also a paradigm that demonstrates that the Alkaline Diet is not just another fad diet, similar to a number of other diets that we will not name. The Alkaline Diet is founded on the comprehension of the significance of pH in maintaining health and preventing the development of diseases in the future. Despite the fact that many people around the world will develop osteoporosis through no fault of their own, there are steps you can take to prevent or at least delay the onset of this dreaded condition if you are approaching old age.

One of the ways in which your body helps to maintain a homeostatic pH is by preparing soluble substances from various parts of the body to elevate the pH, with bone being one of these areas. If you are as of now assisting your body with being more alkaline, you diminish the danger of your body preparing an unresolved issue with the pH of the blood, and you also encourage the body to store bone instead of separating. This is a confidential Alkaline Diet document. This diet can drive the body towards bone consolidation rather than bone loss.

The Alkaline Diet can initiate weight loss because "antacid debris" food sources are typically lower in calories than corrosive debris food sources and frequently include healthy antioxidants. Although the primary goal of a weight-watcher on the Alkaline Diet is typically not weight loss, you can help push your body towards weight loss by consuming food sources that contain the correct proportion of 80% basic debris sources and 20% corrosive debris sources. Again, what's remarkable about this diet is that it has a large number of surprising advantages that the majority of calorie counters did not consider when they decided to begin this diet. You may have started the Alkaline Diet with the hope that it would prevent you from developing the painful kidney stones that run in your family. However, you've also noticed that your skin has improved, your hair is thicker and shinier, you've lost some of that stubborn stomach fat, and you may have even increased your life expectancy. To say "No" to all of these, you would have to be a complete idiot. Before beginning any diet, it is essential to create a list of the goals you hope to achieve. This will both encourage you to stick to your diet when times are tough and help you determine if you are making the expected progress on your diet.

This is a mystery that pertains to all diets, but it is especially pertinent to this one because, for a great many of you, your goal may not be weight loss alone.

The benefit of having weight loss as an objective is that it should be relatively simple to determine whether or not you are achieving it, right? You weigh yourself after one week, two weeks, three weeks, etc., and should be able to quantify whether or not you are losing weight. As many people on this diet will have other motivations for choosing it over others, it will be essential for you to monitor whether or not you are achieving these objectives. This is not only for practical reasons: what's the purpose of going to the farmer's market twice a week to buy pomegranates and wheatgrass if you have no idea if the diet is working because you can't remember why you started it?

Don 't misunderstand me. In view of the fact that you need to maintain a healthy lifestyle, it is perfectly acceptable to continue following a strict diet. In all honesty, this is one of the best reasons to avoid junk cuisine. But if you had specific reasons for choosing this diet, it would be essential to record them in some way, wouldn't it? This is the essential to success on any diet.

Mixed Vegetable Potpie

Easy   **cook**
 INGREDIENTS:

- 5-10 garlic cloves, finely chopped
- 4 cups vegetable broth
- 2 tsp. dried oregano
- 1-3 tsps. sea salt
- 2 bay leaf
- Pinch red pepper flakes
- 2 all-purpose pie crust
- Cooking spray
- 2 large carrot, peeled and finely chopped
- 2 large sweet potato, peeled and chopped into 1inch pieces 2 medium onion, finely chopped
- 2 celery stalk, finely chopped
- ¼ cup chopped broccoli florets (optional)
- 2 large shiitake mushroom, or 8 to 10 white mushrooms, chopped ⅓ cup frozen peas

DIRECTIONS:

1. Preheat the oven to 350°F(2 80°C). Use cooking spray to spray a medium skillet.
2. Add the carrot, sweet potato, onion, celery, broccoli, mushrooms, peas, and garlic. Sauté over medium heat for 10 minutes, or until slightly softened.

3. Stir in the broth, oregano, salt, bay leaf, and red pepper flakes.
4. Simmer the mixture for about 10 minutes, or until thickened and bubbly.
5. Remove from the heat and allow to cool   slightly.

6. Evenly divide the vegetable mixture among four individual ramekins.

7. Roll the pie dough to a 1/2 inch thickness.
8. Easy cut the dough into circles larger than   the   ramekins   slightly.

9. Top one dough disc of each ramekin.

10.   Press the edges down to seal.

11.   Easy cut an opening in the top with a sharp knife to let steam escape while cooking. Arrange the filled ramekins on a baking sheet. Bake for 25 to 30 minutes.

12.   Remove from the oven and let cool slightly. Serve warm.

Carrot Ginger Soup

Ingredients

2 tsp tasteless vegetable oil
2 00 ml coconut milk
100 ml freshly squeezed orange juice
salt
1200g of carrots
2 potato
4 cm grated fresh ginger
2 small onion

Preparation:

1. Clean the carrots and easy cut them into slices. Peel the potatoes and easy cut them into small pieces.
2. Finely chop the onion.
3. Fry the onion in oil until translucent, then add the carrots, ginger and potatoes, roast them briefly and pour in water - don't use too much, it should just cover the vegetables well.
4. Salt to taste.
5. Easy cook the vegetables until soft, add the coconut milk and continue to simmer for 5-10 minutes.
6. Mash the vegetables and stir in the orange juice.
7. Boil briefly again.
8. If the soup is too thick, add a little water and boil again.

Tangy Lentil Soup

☐ 6 cloves chive, finely chopped
☐ 1/2   teaspoon ground turmeric
☐ Sea salt, to taste
☐ Topping
☐ 1/2   cup coconut yogurt
☐ 4 cups red lentils, picked over and rinsed
☐ 2 serrano Chile pepper, chopped
☐ 2 large tomato, chopped, roughly
☐ 1-5 -inch piece ginger, peeled and grated

DIRECTIONS:

1. Add lentils to a pot and with enough water to cover it.
2. Bring the lentils to a boil then reduce the heat.
3. Easy cook for 20 minutes on low simmer.

4. Stir in all the remaining ingredients. Easy cook until lentils are soft and well mixed.
5. Garnish a dollop of coconut yogurt. Serve.

CONCLUSION

Alkaline diets result in a more alkaline urine ph and may reduce the amount of sodium in the urine. However, in some recent studies, this does not reflect the total sodium balance because of other buffers, such as rhodorhate. There is no convincing evidence that osteoporosis improves bone health or prevents fractures. However, alkaline diets have a number of health benefits, as described below.Increased fruits and vegetables in an alkaline diet would increase the K/Na ratio and may improve bone health, reduce muscle waste, and mitigate other sarcoma-related conditions. Please ush a hurertenon and troke. The resultant increase in growth hormone with an alkaline diet may enhance a variety of outcomes, including sardine health, memory, and cognition. An increase in intracellular magnesium, which is required for the function of many enzymes, is an additional advantage of an alkaline diet. Available magnesium, which is required for vitamin D activation, would result in numerous additional benefits for the vitamin D apocrine/exocrine system. Alkalntu may result in additional benefits for some shemotheraphy agents requiring a higher rH. From the evidence presented above, it would be imprudent to infer the presence of an alkali. Reduce the incidence and mortality of swine diseases that are ravaging our aging population. One of the first considerations in an alkaline diet, which includes more fruits and vegetables, is the type of soil in which they were grown, as this can significantly affect the mineral content. Currently, there are a limited number of studies in this field, and many more are needed to examine muscle efficacy, growth hormone, and vitamin D supplementation.

Staunchly humidify and wsh uour drinking water

We are all aware that remaining hydrated is essential, but how safe is your drinking water? In many countries and regions around the world, tar water contains contaminants and cancer-causing compounds, which can deteriorate our health over time. Did you know that changing your drinking water can have a significant impact on your health and energy levels? The most effective way to alkalize water is with a water ionizer machine, which produces water with a rH that you can drink and filters out toxins, metals, and particles. This may be an expensive option for some, so I recommend choosing spring water whenever possible (keep in mind that a lot of bottled water is essentially tar water, so read labels) or drinking filtered tap water (countertop or under-sink water flter) to remove as many contaminants as possible. Even if you only have access to municipal water, it is always vitally important to stay hydrated.

Get more exercise

Phusal astvtu is essential for the human body as we know it. Many of us have sedentary lifestyles, moving from our beds to our chairs to our workstations to our couches when we return home. Rinse. Repeat. All it takes is to move more. Consider taking a dance lesson or participating in your favorite activity on a more consistent basis. Take up running, walking, or whatever else strikes your fancy.

Avoid plastic

It may seem harmless to purchase food in plastic containers, to store leftovers in plastic containers, and to drink from plastic water bottles, but by doing so, we are actually affecting our body's pH levels and causing numerous health problems. Plastic actually resembles estrogen, interfering with your endocrine system and causing havoc, illness, and infertility. The best option is to replace as many plastics in your home with glass or stainless steel alternatives, including water bottles, lunch boxes, and storage containers.

By adhering to these simple lifestyle tips, you are taking a significant step toward healing your body and restoring its pH balance. In addition, your mental health and contentment will improve, which will have a positive effect on your child's development.
Nearing the end of the book, you should feel inspired and motivated to make the necessary adjustments in your life to improve your health, happiness, and overall well-being. But first, I would like to share with you the most important tips and techniques you need to know before embarking on this journey so that you are set up for success and not failure.

No matter your age, birth control pills and synthetic hormone replacement therapy are bad news. Not only are they extremely toxic to your entire body and highly addictive, but they also interact with your endocrinology system, producing synthetic hormones that only prolong your suffering and disrupt your body's natural balance. There are many gentler options for preventing unintended pregnancies, relieving menstrual symptoms, and treating acne than taking synthetic hormones.

Recipes for Alkaline Diet

Alkaline Juices, Smoothies, Tea, and Tons

Alkalizing Fresh Juise Resires

Your dailu multivitamin has never tasted better. Frech juse offer a plethora of health benefits and are vastly superior to the low-nutrient, preserved juse available at your local urermarket.
Vital for optimal health is optimal hydration, and these juices will help you achieve that and more. Due to the fact that juicing removes the fiber from

fruits and vegetables, it is a fantastic way to help you assimilate and absorb nutrients with less digestive effort. Juices contain eental electrolytes, rhutoshemsal, vtamn and mneral - are highly alkalizing, full of antioxdant, and are a great way to consume additional vegetables without having to chew them.

For maximum taste and health benefits, it is best to drink juises within thirtu minutes of being made - though if uou're in a rinsh, uou san rlase juises in an airtight container to avoid oxidization (glass jars work excellent) and store in the refrigerator.

Veggie Stick & Hummous

INGREDIENT :

• For the hummus:

• 2 clove garlic

- Lemon juice of the half lemon
- 2 tbsp olive oil
- 2 can of dried chickpeas, soaked
- 2 tbsp tahini

- For the sticks:
- 2 pepper (green, red, or yellow)
- 1 cucumber
- 2 celery stick
- 2 carrot

•

Combine the legumes and another ingredient using a hand mixer. Using crushed black pepper and Himalayan salt, season to taste.

• For a distinct flavor profile, add fresh tomatoes or chilies just before mixing.

• For the sticks: • Thinly slice all vegetables to create spears long enough to hold a substantial amount of dip but short enough to be easily handled.

Carrot and pepper are blended into oat patties.

Ingredients

2 tsp paprika powder
1 tsp salt
1 tsp chilli flakes
1 tsp garlic powder
250 g oat flakes
200 g carrots
1 Paprika
2 red onion
200 ml water

Preparation:

1. First, peel the carrot and then grate it finely.
2. Then peel the onion and easy cut it into small pieces together with the pepper.

3. Put the vegetables in a large bowl and add the oat flakes.

4. Then add the spices and mix everything well.

5. Then add the water and stir everything. Now leave to infuse for at least 25 to 30 minutes.

6. Then, wet your hands and shape the mixture into about 15 fritters.

7. Heat a little oil in a pan and fry the patties on both sides until they are nice and crispy.

Easy Chia Pudding Recipe

Ingredients

- 4 Tbsp chia seeds
- 1 cup almond or cashew milk
- 1 tsp honey or maple syrup
- vanilla

To top:
- berries
- 2 tsp almond butter
- chopped nuts (optional)

Instructions

1. Place chia seeds, honey or maple syrup vanilla and liquid of choice in a jar with a lid.
2. Stir with a fork until the chia seeds aren't clumping anymore.
3. Cover with the lid and refrigerate overnight.
4. Top with berries, a tsp of almond butter and optionally coconut or chopped nuts.

Vegan Instant Pot Cabbage Detox Soup

Ingredients

2 onion, chopped
4 cloves garlic
4 tablespoons apple cider vinegar
2 tablespoon lemon juice
4 teaspoons dried sage
6 cups coarsely chopped green cabbage
5 cups vegetable broth
2 (2 8 .10 ounce) can diced tomatoes
6 carrots, chopped
6 stalks celery, chopped

Directions

1. Combine cabbage, vegetable broth, diced tomatoes, carrots, celery, onion, garlic, apple cider vinegar, lemon juice, and sage in a multi-functional pressure cooker.
2. Close and lock the lid.
3. Select high pressure according to manufacturer's instructions; set timer for 25 to 30 minutes.

4. Allow 2 0 to 2 10 minutes for pressure to build.
5. Release pressure using the natural-release method according to manufacturer's instructions, 70 to 80 minutes.
6. Unlock and remove lid.

Lettuce, Zucchini And Hummus Wrap

INGREDIENTS:

- 8 tbsps. of homemade hummus
- 2 cup of romaine lettuce
- 2 sliced plum tomato
- ½ sliced red onion
- 2 tbsp. of grape seed oil
- 2 sliced zucchini
- Pure sea salt, to taste
- Cayenne, to taste
- 4 tortillas

DIRECTIONS:

• Warm the grape seed oil in a grill pan over medium heat.

• Add the zucchini slices to the pan and season with the sea salt and cayenne pepper.

• Cook Easy cook on medium heat for approximately 5-10 minutes, then rotate and cook for an additional 1-5 minutes. Take it off the burner.

• Place each tortilla on the grill and cook for 1-5 minutes on low heat until heated.

• Take off the barbecue.

• Fill the center of each tortilla with two tablespoons of homemade hummus, lettuce, onion, tomato, and zucchini segments.

• Securely wrap and serve.

Broccoli Soup

Ingredients for 2 servings:
leftover stem parts of broccoli stems and some florets

2 tsp garlic powder
2 clove of garlic, finely chopped
4 tbsp fresh cress
2 potato
2 small onion, finely chopped
2 tsp olive oil
2 tsp onion powder
Salt pepper

Preparation:

The broccoli stems and potato should be peeled and then cut into tiny pieces.
Cook the onion in oil before adding the garlic.
Pour approximately 5-10 milliliter of water into the pan and add the sliced vegetables.
Allow the broth to simmer on low for approximately twenty minutes.
When the broccoli and potato are fully cooked, pulverize them with a hand blender.
Season with onion and garlic powder, salt and pepper, and garnish with fresh cress before serving.

LENTIL KALE SOUP

vegetable broth powder, 2 teaspoon, dried
Sazon seasoning, 2 teaspoon
red lentils, 2 cup
Seville orange juice, 2 tablespoon
alkaline water, 6 cups
2 bunch kale
 Onion, 1
Zucchinis, 4
Celery, 2 rib
  Chive, 2 stalk
tomatoes, 2 cup, diced

DIRECTIONS:

1. Add all the vegetables to a greased pan.
2. Sauté for 10   minutes then add broth, tomatoes, and Sazon seasoning.

3. Mix well and stir in red lentils along with   water.

4. Easy cook until lentil is soft and tender.
5. Add kale and easy cook for minutes.
6. Serve warm with Seville orange slices on top.

GARLIC DRESSING

- 4 tbsp of avocado oil
- Himalayan salt
- Black pepper
- 2 clove garlic
- 2 lemon

DIRECTIONS :

1. Smash the garlic clove, then combine lemon juice, avocado oil, and spices in a small bowl.

2. Serving with a salad or other vegetables once the infusion has finished for 15 mins is recommended.
   How much lemon juice and olive oil you use is up to you?

Savoru Avocado Wrap

Ingredients:

2 tsp. cilantro, chopped
½ red onion, diced
2 tomato, sliced or chopped
Sea salt & pepper
2 butter lettuce or collard leaf bunch
1 haas avocado
2 tsp. chopped basil
Small handful of spinach

Directions:
1. Spread avocado onto leaf and sprinkle with basil, cilantro, red onion, tomato, salt and pepper and add spinach. Fold in half and enjoy!

Vegetable curry made with fresh coriander.

Ingredients

1 tsp ground turmeric
1000 ml vegetable stock
500 ml coconut milk
60 g fresh coriander
Squeeze of fresh lime juice
1400 g Hokkaido pumpkin
800 g waxy potatoes
400 g carrots
400 g onions
4 cloves garlic
60 g ginger
4 small red chillies
4 tbsp roasted sesame oil
A little salt

Preparation:

First, thoroughly wash and dry the pumpkin before cutting it into tiny cubes. Additionally, peel the potatoes and carrots and dice them into tiny cubes.

Now, peel the onions, ginger, and garlic, then dice them into small pieces. Then, wash the peppers and finely slice them.

In a heated saucepan, briefly sweat the onions and garlic in oil.

Then, add the carrots, pumpkin, and potatoes. Now, quickly sauté everything, but do not neglect to stir.

Grilled Macrobiotic Bowl

Ingredients

• salt and pepper to taste
Garlic Cashew Creme
• 1 cup raw cashews
• 6 cloves garlic
• 1 teaspoon sea salt
• juice of 2 lemon
• 4 tablespoon olive oil
• 4 tablespoon garlic, minced
• 1 cup cubed butternut squash
• 2 cup cooked brown rice or quinoa I used Seeds of Change Brown Rice and Quinoa
• 1 cup sauerkraut
• 1 cup adzuki beans cooked
• 1 cup baby kale or your preferred greens
• 2 tablespoon dulse flakes
• 2 tablespoon toasted pumpkin seeds

Instructions

1. Pre easy cook butternut in microwave for 1-5 minutes
2. Spread olive oil on grill. *See notes if you are not grilling.
3. Add butternut, rice, beans, greens, sauerkraut, to the grill.
4. Grill on medium high for 15 to 20 minutes, turning frequently until done. Salt and pepper to taste.
5. Assemble bowl
6. Sprinkle dulse flakes and toasted pumpkin seeds
7. Top with Garlic Cashew Creme

Turkey Burgers Stuffed with Bread, Cranberries, and Fresh Rosemary

Ingredients

½ cup dried cranberries, chopped
4 ounces Brie cheese, cubed
4 tablespoons tomato ketchup
4 sprigs fresh rosemary, chopped
salt and pepper to taste
2   slice white bread, torn into small
pieces
2 clove garlic, minced
6 tablespoons boiling water
2 pound ground turkey
1 medium red onion, chopped

Minimalist Melon & Lemon Wonder

Ingredients

Mint to garnish (optional)
Watermelon, 4 cups
1 lemon, peeled

Direction

1. Chop and de-seed watermelon and press through your juicer, along with lemon.
2. Juice, garnish and ready to take

Citrus, Sweet Potato, and Lime Creamsicle

Ingredients

8 fresh carrots, ends trimmed
2 raw medium sweet potato, peeled
4 medium oranges
2 lime

Direction

1. Peel the oranges, lime and sweet potato. Top and tail the carrots.
2. Add all of the ingredients to your juicer.
3. Juice and ready to take

www.ingramcontent.com/pod-product-compliance
Lightning Source LLC
Chambersburg PA
CBHW060653030426
42337CB00017B/2592